Poisons of the Intelligence

Charles Richet
Virgil G. Eaton

Poisons of the Intelligence :

Hasheesh, Opium and other Narcotics

LM Publishers

Poisons of the Intelligence : the Hasheesh[1]

Hasheesh is the extract of Indian hemp. This extract, mixed with different aromatics and vegetable oils, forms *dawamesk*, a sort of nauseous confection taken before a meal. Then there is the hasheesh smoked in pipes or in cigarettes, and this is the form in which the drug is most commonly taken in the East. The aqueous extract is known as *hafioun;* it is more active than the other two preparations. It takes nearly four parts of dawamesk to make one of hafioun. It is very difficult to find out any more concerning the Oriental modes of preparing hasheesh; still, though our pharmaceutical information be insufficient, we are pretty

[1] By Charles Richet

familiar with the psychic effects of the drug. I have taken it myself again and again in various doses, and have administered it to many of my friends, and whatever I shall have to say concerning its properties will be based upon my own observations. Taken in moderate doses, it produces a kind of intoxication that is very pleasant, highly advantageous for a correct knowledge of intellectual phenomena, and at the same time free from serious consequences. The worst that is to be expected when one takes either dawamesk or hafioun in suitable quantities is slight disorder of the digestion, and a little sense of heaviness and of cerebral excitation.

If one has not been told what to expect, the first effects of hasheesh pass by unnoticed; these consist of a certain motor and sensor excitability of the spinal cord. There is a twitching in the nape of the neck, the back and the legs, and a shivering that extends over the whole body. It is as though there were puffs of hot and cold air rising to the head; but withal there is a vague sense of comfortableness, and one finds himself in a state of great good-humor, as is the case of most persons after the absorption of a certain amount of alcohol. By degrees the excitation of the spinal cord produces effects that are more characteristic, as muscular exertion of every kind, walking, stretching, dancing, lifting heavy weights; but meantime the mind is calm. Suddenly, however, on hearing some chance remark, the patient is seized with a fit of laughing without any apparent cause, and this continues for a length of time. This having passed, he comes to himself again, and recognizes the first effects of the poison.

Ideas now come crowding on his brain, one following another with bewildering rapidity. Thoughts come and go without any apparent law of succession or concomitance, but in reality they are governed by the immutable laws of the association of ideas and impressions. The patient thinks the persons he sees around him very slow and dull. Language is not swift enough to give expression to his rapid thoughts. There is, as it were, an hypertrophy of ideas. What in the normal state would cause very trifling discomfort, now becomes an unbearable evil, and the patient cries and begs for commiseration. With the air of a tragic actor he will tell you that it rains, or that the wind blows. One's self-esteem is magnified, and he looks down with scorn upon the ignorance of others.

Thus, then, to say nothing as yet of the change in sensation, the moral person is entirely transformed. I am not aware that the resemblance of these phenomena to those of hysteria has ever been noticed. In general, hysterical women are very intelligent, with brilliant ideas and a lively imagination; but their mental activity labors under two defects, namely, the exaggeration of the feelings and the absence of will. The same thing is seen in the use of hasheesh.

But there are other phenomena that are still more characteristic of hasheesh, especially its effects on our notions of time and space. Under its influence, time seems to be of interminable length. Between two clearly-conceived ideas the patient descries a host of others that are indeterminate and incomplete, and of which he is only dimly conscious; but he is filled with admiration at their number and vastness. Now we measure time by the memory of the ideas that have passed through the mind, and hence an instant appears immensely long to one under the hasheesh influence. Suppose, as is common enough in the use of this drug, that in the space of one second fifty different thoughts enter the brain; now, since in the normal state it requires several minutes to conceive fifty different thoughts, the inference will be that many minutes have gone by. Seconds become years, and minutes become ages.

This illusion has no parallel; yet in dreaming, or rather in that intermediate state which is neither sleeping nor waking, we experience something similar. I recollect having been at work one day with a friend, and, as I felt drowsy, asking him to let me sleep for a few minutes. On awaking, I was assured by him that I had slept hardly a second; and yet in that brief time I had had a very complicated dream, and, in consequence of the multiplicity of my thoughts, the time had appeared to be of considerable length. So, if a person be awakened by some sudden, loud noise, he will oftentimes, in the fraction of a second, pass in imagination through scenes and adventures of a very complicated nature. A like illusion may be procured at will by shutting the eyes while one is riding in a carriage: under such circumstances the journey will appear to have no end; on opening the eyes from time to time, and observing the landmarks, the progress will seem to be extremely slow.

But in dreaming and in sleep this illusion as to the lapse of time is vague and ill-defined. Under the influence of hasheesh, on the contrary, it becomes singularly definite. Nor is the illusion of the sight less astonishing, which causes inconsiderable distances to appear enormously great. I do not know whether this illusion has been observed under any other conditions than those of hasheesh-poisoning, nor can I offer any rational explanation of it. It is difficult even to describe it. It causes a bridge, an avenue, to stretch out to unheard-of lengths. On going up a ladder, the rounds appear to reach up to the sky. A river whose opposite bank is in sight becomes an arm of the sea. And, besides these two illusions of space and time, which by-the-way often persist twenty-four hours or more, there are other illusions of the strangest kind imaginable. Hallucinations, on the contrary, are infrequent, though one remarkable instance has been observed by Dr. Moreau, of Tours.

It is oftentimes very hard to draw the distinction between illusion and hallucination, but nevertheless there is a difference between these two manifestations of morbid psychic activity. When an insane patient sees at his elbow a walking, talking spectre, he has an hallucination. But if in a dark forest, at night, one takes some deformed trunk for a ghost, he has an illusion. Illusion presupposes an actual sensation, the perception of which is exaggerated and erroneous, whereas hallucination comes spontaneously without requiring a sensation to give rise to it. Now, under the hasheesh influence, the sensations are exaggerated so as to produce endless illusions. The slightest sound becomes a crash, and we hear the fall of waters, the roar of cataracts, the blare of trumpets, or brilliant harmonies. I have seen persons, naturally almost insensible to music, lifted by a few musical notes into an ecstasy such as we read of in the lives of saints. But, for a description of all these sensations, I would refer the reader to the brilliant pages of Théophile Gautier's "Club des Hachichins."

I will not go over ground trod by Gautier, but will content myself with touching upon another point of psychological interest. We will suppose the illusion to be stronger than anything noticed in the foregoing instances; that instead of being a simple disorder of the perceptive faculties, it affects the conceptive powers. Under normal conditions, external impressions awaken manifold ideas in our minds; besides the association of ideas, there is association of impressions with ideas. For instance, a certain taste, smell, or sound, gives rise to a multitude of conceptions that follow one another according to the direction we may be pleased to give them. The faculty of attention enables us to check the uprising of the conceptions called forth by the taste, smell, or sound. Often, while attention is fixed on an object, we neither hear nor see what is passing without. In reality we do see and hear, but these sensations are obliterated, and pass out of the mind without leaving a trace behind. In the use of hasheesh, in virtue of the loss of will, the intensity of the perceptions, and the excitation of the brain, every external impression calls forth a series of delirious conceptions, and there is no check.

Dr. Moreau lays great stress on the resemblance subsisting between these hasheesh illusions and the systematic delirium of the insane. In most lunatics the delirious idea has its origin in fact, in a sensation, a pain, an impression from without. This forms for them the logical basis of a system of erroneous judgments. If, for instance, they suffer from nausea or gastric pains, they say they have been poisoned; that their enemies have mixed poison with their food. Precisely the same thing is found in the use of hasheesh. Every sensation immediately calls forth an insane thought, or rather a thousand such thoughts. Hence it really appears as though the veil were rent in twain, and that by the use of this drug we are enabled to witness the mind itself at its work. The mysterious and silent travail which in the normal state produces our thoughts and judgments is no longer either mysterious or silent: we can see how the whole is connected, and can look on while ideas are being evolved. But, unfortunately, under the hasheesh influence one is no longer master of his own thoughts, and must, perforce, follow them in their disorderly course. Here we observe close resemblance between the three states of dreaming, insanity, and hasheesh intoxication. In all these external impressions are all-powerful, and the mind is subject, unchecked, to the excitation of the senses.

One great difference between intoxication by hasheesh and that by alcohol and chloroform is that in the former, when the dose is light, memory is intact: one remembers with marvelous exactitude all that he saw, did, or said. But if the dose be strong, the loss of memory is complete; then, too, there is delirium, wild delirium. In such doses hasheesh is dangerous, though I do not think a single case of death from this cause has ever been recorded in Europe. But sometimes the delirium has continued for several days, and assumed serious proportions. No one should take hasheesh without having some person to care for him while under the influence of the drug; oftentimes the hasheesh gives such a sense of lightness and agility that a person will attempt to fly by leaping out of a window.

In the East hasheesh is in very general use. It is nearly always smoked in large pipes, which are passed from mouth to mouth. The smoke is very agreeable, possessing a peculiar aromatic odor. On entering certain Arab *cafés* at Cairo or at Damascus, one perceives this penetrating odor, which gently intoxicates even those who do not smoke. In this mild dose hasheesh produces a sort of sleepiness, during which external objects assume fantastic forms, and all is like a dream. The monotonous, nasal music has a gentle, tranquilizing effect during this sleep. On the walls of the *café* are rudely-pictured camels, grotesque human forms, or the surface is marked with lines, quadrangles, and triangles. In the minds of the hasheesh-smokers these rude pictures awaken delightful illusions, and they fancy themselves to be transported to Mohammed's paradise. To further amuse the indolence of the customers, a chanter drones out a long story, semi-religious, semi-heroic. The tale is in couplets, and between the couplets the music strikes up again its interminable rhythm. Now and then a smoker will rise staggering to his feet, and will give expression by yells to the delight with which he contemplates some fantastic image that he sees. The rest of the company then laugh uproariously, but anon will greet the last speaker with "Allah be with thee! Allah be praised!" Never shall I forget this spectacle, which, in a dark corner of the noisy bazaars of Damascus, with the dim light of a smoky lamp, to the sound of the tambourine and guitar with three cords, enabled me to understand one side of Oriental life.

Poisons of the Intelligence : Chloroform

Chloroform is a colorless, volatile, oily liquid; it is denser than water, and does not mix with it. It was discovered by Soubeiran in 1831, and Soubeiran's process for obtaining it is still in use, viz., distilling alcohol with calcium hypochlorite and lime. The hypnotic properties of chloroform were discovered in 1847 by Flourens, a few months after Jackson had recognized similar properties in ether; but the first surgeon who made use of it in an operation on the human subject was Simpson, of Edinburgh, in November, 1847. Since then, the use of chloroform has become so general, that nowadays no great operation in surgery is attempted without employing it. We may, therefore, justly regard the discovery of surgical anæsthesia as one of the greatest scientific achievements of the present century, so fruitful of benefits to the human race.

The principal effect of chloroform is the paralysis of sensibility, or anæsthesia. In so far forth it acts upon the mind, for sensibility is only one of the forms of mind; but this point, which as yet is rather obscure, calls for a few words of explanation.

Two great functions devolve upon the nervous system, sensibility and motion: it is through sensibility that we receive impressions from without; and it is through the excitation of the muscles, or movement, that we manifest our will, or act upon external objects. In the absence of both disease and poisoning, the will—that is, the mind—excites, through the spinal cord, the various muscles, producing movement; but this condition is not absolutely necessary, since in decapitated animals, for instance, the nervous system of the spinal cord can of itself produce motion of the muscles. Here we have motor activity, but no sensibility. Sensibility exists only where the mind is intact and capable of perceiving, so that a creature which has no mind is void of sensibility. This fact is confirmed by pathological observation; for, whenever the mind is affected, there appear at the same time symptoms of disordered sensibility, and *vice versa*. And when we find a patient exhibiting notable disorder of the sensibility, then, if the nerves are intact, we can safely conclude that the central nervous system is affected, and to that degree that the mind has not escaped.

Anatomy and physiology here are in accord with pathology. Some animals possess little or no sensibility: they belong to the lower grades of animals; their intelligence is obscure, and their sensibility is as obtuse as their intelligence. On the other hand, if we consider animals of higher intelligence, we find their sensibility becoming more and more keen, till we come to man, at once the most intelligent and the most sensitive of animals. And even in man himself we find race differences, those races being most sensitive which possess the highest decree of intelligence. The anatomical structure of the nervous centres is in harmony with this coincidence, for it is in man that the posterior columns of the spinal cord are most voluminous, as compared with the anterior. Now, the anterior columns transmit the motor excitations to the nerves, while the posterior columns transmit the sensory excitations. Again, the posterior lobes of the brain in man, as compared with animals, are more developed than the anterior. But it is in the posterior lobes that perception of sensitive excitations appears to reside.

Nor is it surprising that there should exist so intimate a relation between mind and sensibility. Indeed, whatever may be the influence of the spontaneous development of the mind itself, resulting from the constitution of the brain, which is its organ, it still holds true that all our knowledge comes from our sensations, and from the brain-work thence resulting. Mind is, so to speak, the product of these two factors; and our notions of the world around us, elaborated and fecundated by the mind's spontaneous action, constitute individual personality. Hence, inasmuch as anatomy, physiology, and pathology, show intimate relation between sensibility and intelligence, we can justly say that psychology confirms the positive data furnished by these three sciences.

Accordingly, poisons which affect the intelligence are *ipso facto* poisons of the sensibility. In this respect alcohol does not differ from chloroform. When alcoholic intoxication is only beginning, we find already a notable degree of insensibility; but at the comatose stage the insensibility is total, just as in the last stage of chloroform. Thus intoxication by chloroform and intoxication by alcohol proceed along parallel lines, and we can distinguish a first period of intoxication, properly so called, and a second period of sleep or coma.

When a person takes chloroform, the first few inhalations make him dizzy; he is seized with a sort of vertigo and dimness of vision. This vertigo goes on increasing, and, as the patient continues to respire the toxic agent, his ideas become more and more exalted. He hears what is said to him and makes replies, but he does so after the manner of a drunken man, at first exaggerating his impressions and regardless of proportion. His judgment has already disappeared, and he utters the most insignificant replies with a theatrical accent, the effect being often grotesque. Next, his ideas grow more and more mixed: will and judgment being gone, ideation is disordered and delirious; in short, we have a state of sleep accompanied with dreaming, closely resembling ordinary sleep.

When the chloroform absorbed by the mucous membrane of the lungs has passed into the blood, *active* memory, which presupposes attention and will, has disappeared; still, the intelligence is not yet dead. Ideas are still conceived, old recollections persist, and sometimes even the memory of past events is strangely quickened. The patient will speak in a language he thought he had forgotten, and recall old stories that seemed to have passed into oblivion. This superexcitation of memory is all the more interesting because in sundry forms of mental alienation it occurs with the same characters—these, too, being accompanied by entire loss of *active* memory.

Though insensibility supervenes very soon after the administration of chloroform, commonly it occurs only after the loss of memory, and this circumstance leads to very singular results. Thus, if the surgeon begins the operation before perfect insensibility has been produced, the patient will cry out, and beg to have it delayed till the drug has had full influence. One might suppose, from his cries of pain and his contortions, that the chloroform had produced no effect, and yet on awaking he has no recollection of what has taken place.

Is that real pain which leaves in the mind no trace? The answer to this question is not so easy as one might imagine. Suppose an acute, penetrating pain, continuing only for about one minute. Undoubtedly the patient suffers real pain during that minute; but, if all memory of it disappeared at once, then the patient would deny that he had suffered at all, and would not hesitate to undergo the operation again. In short, he would have enjoyed the benefits of chloroformic anæsthesia.

In administering chloroform, we must take account of the patient's temperament. If he is a resolute, courageous person, all will go on well, and the insensibility will readily disappear; if, on the contrary, he has an unconquerable dread of the operation, great watchfulness will be necessary, for in such cases syncope is very frequent. Besides, such a patient resists the action of the drug for a long time, and it must be administered in far greater quantity than in the other case. The chloroform always retains its power, but the cerebral excitation to which some patients are subject enables them to resist its toxic action, as though the will could, so to speak, brace itself up to resist the action of the poison on the nerve-centres. The same occurs in the use of alcohol. One who *will* not be intoxicated may drink a large quantity without being drunk. At length, however, his will is conquered, and he falls to the ground, but he will not have experienced the exhilaration, the mad excitation, of the man who gives himself up to the influence of the liquor.

Thus, then, under the action of chloroform we find an antagonism existing between the various intellectual faculties—on the one hand the voluntary, and on the other the unconscious faculties. The latter are slowest to disappear; ideation, its guide and check, being deranged or destroyed, follows its habitual laws: association of ideas persists. External sensations are still borne in upon the mind, each one awaking a long series of ideas. As the sense of hearing is the last to disappear, the patient, though he can no longer either see or feel, hears every word that is spoken, and is set a-thinking at once. The same thing occurs in ordinary sleep, rarely in adults, but very frequently in young children. In fact, a certain degree of natural somnambulism is nearly always to be found in children. The child speaks out aloud without waking, he laughs and talks; more frequently he is frightened and cries. The course of his thoughts may be altered, diverted into another channel, by speaking to him gently, and this without arousing him from sleep. On awaking, all recollection of this has vanished. This method has been tried in mental alienation, to divert the thoughts of melancholies and hypochondriacs.

But soon these external phenomena which indicate the preservation of the intelligence, if not its integrity, disappear in their turn. The period of excitation is succeeded by the period of relaxation, and then the patient is in a deep sleep. However violent the external excitations, however painful the surgical operation, nothing can arouse the patient out of the comatose state into which he has fallen. His respiration is regular, his pulse slow and full, his pupils are motionless, and his features, paralyzed as it were, no longer wear that convulsive grimace which may be regarded as the last trace of sensibility. Intelligence is now destroyed. The coma of chloroform and that of alcohol appear to be essentially one. And, yet, what a difference! The former saves man from pain, the latter drags man down to the lowest depths of degradation; yet in both all signs of intellectual life have disappeared—there is a temporary death of the mind. It may be that, in the inmost nerve-tissues, brain-work still goes on, unconscious and silent, but whether this is so we know not.

How the Opium Habit is acquired[2]

I am not one of the persons who raise a great cry about the evils of the "opium-habit." I have no doubt that the continued use of narcotics, whether they be tobacco or opium, is injurious to the nervous system; but I also firmly believe that the recuperative powers of the body are such that they can largely overcome any harmful results coming from the regular use of these substances. For instance, I know a stone-cutter who resides at Cape Elizabeth, Me., who for the past twenty years has used twenty cents' worth of black "navy plug" tobacco every day. He is a large, vigorous man, weighing over two hundred pounds. His

---

[2] By Virgil G. Eaton

appetite is good; he sleeps well, and, save for a little heart disturbance caused by overstimulation, he is perfectly healthy, and is likely to live until he is fourscore. He is now fifty-one years of age, and he assures me he has used tobacco since he was fourteen, and never had a fit of "swearing off" in his life. A peculiar and, I should say, a rather troublesome habit of his, is to go to bed every night with a big "quid" of hard "plug" tobacco between his molars. As this is always gone in the morning, and the pillow shows no traces of the weed, he thinks he chews it and swallows it in his sleep, though he never knows anything about the process.

There is a widow who keeps a lodging-house in Oak Street, Boston, Mass., who takes three drachms of morphia sulphate every day, in three one-drachm doses, morning, noon, and night. When it is remembered that an eighth of a grain is the usual dose for an adult, while two grains are sufficient to kill a man, the amount she takes seems startling. I asked her why she did not try and substitute tobacco, or bromide, or chloral hydrate for morphine, and she said they made her sick, so she could not use them. This woman is sixty years old, very pale and emaciated. Her appetite is poor. She attends to her duties faithfully, however, and is able, with the help of a girl, to carry on a large lodging-house.

I might give scores of instances similar to the above, but these will do for my purpose. I believe that the person who takes liquor or tobacco or opium, in regular quantities at stated intervals, is able to withstand their effect after getting fixed in the habit, and that it is the irregular, spasmodic use of these articles which brings delirium and death. It is the man who goes on a "spree," and then quits for a time, who has the weak stomach and aching head. His neighbor, who takes his regular toddy and has his usual smoke, feels no inconvenience.

For the past year or more I have studied the growth of the opium-habit in Boston. It is increasing rapidly. Not only are there more Chinese "joints" and respectable resorts kept by Americans than there were a year ago, but the number of individuals who "hit the pipe" at home and in their offices is growing very fast. A whole opium "lay-out," including pipe, fork, lamp, and spoon, can now be had for less than five dollars. This affords a chance for those who have acquired the habit to follow their desires in private, without having to reveal their secret to anyone. How largely this is practiced I do not know, but, judging from the tell-tale pallor of the faces I see, I feel sure the habit is claiming more slaves every day.

In order to approximate to the amount of opium in its various forms which is used in Boston, I have made a thorough scrutiny of the physicians' recipes left at the drug-stores to be filled. As is well known, all recipes given by physicians are numbered, dated, and kept on file at the drug-stores, so that they may be referred to at any time. To these I went in search of information.

I was surprised to learn how extensively opium and its alkaloids—particularly sulphate of morphia — are used by physicians. I found them prescribed for every ailment which flesh is heir to. They are used for headache, sore eyes, toothache, sore throat. laryngitis, diphtheria, bronchitis, congestion, pneumonia, consumption, gastritis, liver-complaint, stone in the gall-duct, carditis, aneurism, hypertrophy, peritonitis, calculus, kidney trouble, rheumatism, neuralgia, and all general or special maladies of the body. It is the great panacea and cure-all.

During my leisure time I have looked up more than 10,000 recipes. It has been my practice to go to the files, open the book, or take up a spindle at random, and take 300 recipes just as they come. The first store I visited I found 43 recipes which contained morphine out of the 300 examined. Close by, a smaller store, patronized by poorer people, had 36. Up in the aristocratic quarters, where the customers call in carriages, I found 49 morphine recipes in looking over 300. At the North End, among the poor Italian laborers, the lowest proportion of 32 in 300 was discovered. Without detailing all the places visited, I will summarize by saying that, in 10,200 recipes taken in 34 drug-stores, I found 1,481 recipes which prescribed some preparation of opium, or an average of fourteen and one half per cent of the whole.

This was surprising enough; but my investigations did not end here. Of the prescriptions furnished by physicians I found that forty-two per cent were filled the second time, and of those refilled twenty-three per cent contained opium in some form. Again, twenty-eight per cent of all prescriptions are filled a third time; and of these, sixty-one per cent were for opiates; while of the twenty per cent taken for the fourth filling, seventy-eight per cent were for the narcotic drug, proving, beyond a doubt, that it was the opiate qualities of the medicine that afforded relief and caused the renewal.

From conversation with the druggists, I learned that the proprietary or "patent" medicines which have the largest sales were those containing opiates. One apothecary told me of an old lady who formerly came to him as often as four times a week and purchased a fifty-cent bottle of "cough-balsam." She informed him that it "quieted her nerves" and afforded rest when everything else had failed. After she had made her regular visits for over a year, he told her one day that he had sold out of the medicine required, and suggested a substitute, which was a preparation containing about the same amount of morphine. On trial, the woman found the new mixture answered every purpose of the old. The druggist then told her she had acquired the morphine-habit, and from that time on she was a constant morphine-user.

It was hard to learn just what proportion of those who began by taking medicines containing opiates became addicted to the habit. I should say, from what I learned, that the number was fully twenty-five per cent — perhaps more. The proportion of those who, having taken up the habit in earnest, left it off later on, was very small—not over ten per cent. When a person once becomes an opium-slave, the habit usually holds through life.

I was told many stories about the injurious effects of morphine and opium upon the morals of those who use it. One peculiarity of a majority is that, whenever a confirmed user of the narcotic obtains credit at the drug-store, he at once stops trading at that place and goes elsewhere. All the druggists know this habit very well, and take pains to guard against it. Whenever a customer asks for credit for a bottle of morphine, the druggist informs him that the store never trusts any one; but if he has no money with him the druggist will gladly give him enough to last a day or two. In this way the druggist keeps his customer, whereas he would have lost his trade if the present had not been made at the time credit was refused.

Of course, I heard much about the irresistible desire which confirmed slaves to the habit have for their delight. There is nothing too degrading for them to do in order to obtain the narcotic. Many druggists firmly believe that a majority of the seemingly motiveless crimes which are perpetrated by reputable people are due to this habit. In pursuit of opium the slaves will resort to every trick and art which human ingenuity can invent. There is a prisoner now confined in the Concord (Mass.) Reformatory who has his opium smuggled in to him in the shape of English walnuts donated by a friend. The friend buys the opium and, opening the walnut-shells, extracts the meat, and fills up the spaces with the gum. Then he sticks the shells together with glue and sends them to the prison.

At present our clergymen, physicians, and reformers are asking for more stringent laws against the sale of these narcotics. The law compelling every person who purchases opium or other poisons to "register," giving his name and place of residence to the druggist, has been in force in Massachusetts for several years, and all this time the sales have increased. No registration law can control the traffic.

The parties who are responsible for the increase of the habit are the physicians who give the prescriptions. In these days of great mental strain, when men take their business home with them and think of it from waking to sleeping, the nerves are the first to feel the effects of overwork. Opium effects immediate relief, and the doctors, knowing this, and wishing to stand well with their patients, prescribe it more and more. Their design is to effect a cure. The result is to convert their patients into opium slaves. The doctors are to blame for so large a consumption of opium, and they are the men who need reforming.

Two means of preventing the spread of the habit suggest themselves to every thoughtful person:

1) Pass a law that no prescriptions containing opium or its preparations can be

filled more than once at the druggist's without having the physician renew it. The extra cost of calling on a doctor when the medicine ran out would deter many poor people from acquiring the habit. Such a law would also make the doctors more guarded in prescribing opiates for trivial ailments. With the law in force, and the druggists guarded by strict registration laws, we could soon trace the responsibility to its proper source, and then, if these safeguards were not enough, physicians could be fined for administering opiates save in exceptional cases.

2) The great preventive to the habit is to keep the body in such a state that it will not require sedatives or stimulants. The young men and women in our cities have too big heads, too small necks, and too flabby muscles. They should forsake medicine, and patronize the gymnasium. Let them develop their muscles

and rest their nerves, and the family doctor, who means well, but who cannot resist the tendency of the age, can take a protracted vacation. Unless something of the kind is done soon, the residents of our American cities will be all opium-slaves.

Opium and its Antidote[3]

Opium is the juice of the poppy, and, as there are many varieties of the poppy, so too are there many kinds of opium; the mode of collecting the juice is, however, always the same. In Egypt, Syria, and India, the three countries which produce opium, a number of semicircular incisions are made in the capsule of the poppy, and the juice which exudes is carefully gathered. This juice, on being dried in the sun, becomes of a dark color, thickens, and forms a brown, firm paste: this is opium. Laudanum is a solution of opium in alcohol and water. Both opium and laudanum are to be regarded as a mixture of several similar but not

---

[3] By Charles Richet

identical substances. Since the time of Derosne (1804) and Robiquet (1817), who first isolated narcotine and morphine, chemists have very carefully investigated the different chemical compounds occurring in opium. Thus they have discovered codeine, narceine, thebaäine, papaverine, and other substances, all of them bases, i. e., bodies that unite with acids to form crystallizable salts.

These bases do not all affect in the same way the organic functions. Thus, narcotine possesses very little or no soporific power: two grammes of it can be injected without perceptible effect, while a centigramme of morphine is quite sufficient to produce therapeutic and physiological results. Thebäine does not cause sleep, and in animals produces convulsions like those caused by strychnine, while morphine in the same dose produces deep comatose sleep. Another curious thing about these opium alkaloids is, that they do not act alike on man and animals, as has been demonstrated by Claude Bernard. Man is specially sensitive to the action of morphine, while thebäine is almost without effect upon his nervous system: animals, on the other hand, feel the effects of morphine only when it is given in large doses, while thebäine is for them a violent poison. So, too, with belladonna, and atropine, its active principle, they are a deadly poison for man, but almost without effect on rabbits: the dose of atropine that would suffice to kill ten men would hardly be enough to kill one rabbit. The difference is not so great with respect to morphine, yet morphine specially affects man; hence in this article we will consider only this one opium alkaloid.

When, in "Le Malade imaginaire," honest *Argan* is asked why opium causes sleep, his artless reply is, "Quia habet proprietatem dormitivam." Nowadays we are not content with this kind of explanation, and some authors have sought for the "dormitive property" of opium in the state of the cerebral circulation; and, though the true cause has not yet been certainly established, still it is something that research has been made.

It is not yet positively decided whether opium produces anæmia or whether it produces congestion of the brain; indeed, we know little more than did *Argan,* namely, that it sets one asleep. This sleep, however, is in some respects different from ordinary sleep. From thirty to sixty minutes after taking opium one feels a slight excitation; there is a general feeling of buoyancy and contentment, soon followed by drowsiness and a state of reverie rather than of dreaming. There is a pleasurable feeling of *abandon,* and an agreeable sense of torpor creeps over the whole frame; the thoughts are like the ever-shifting scenes of a phantasmagoria, on which we passively gaze, without will or effort to alter the series. Still, so long as the intoxication is not deep, such effort is possible. One feels that he is falling asleep, and that if he would but bestir himself he might overcome his drowsiness. But little by little the legs grow heavy, the arms fall to the sides almost powerless, and the weighted eyelids refuse to remain open. A dreamy, rambling sort of thinking still goes on, and there is as yet no sleep; we are still conscious of the world around. We indistinctly hear the tic-tac of the clock and the rumble of passing vehicles, but it is as though, so to speak, another person were listening and not we. The active, conscious *Me* exists no more, and another personality seems to have taken its place. Gradually everything becomes more and more indistinct, our thoughts are enveloped in a haze, we feel ourselves detached from matter, detached from our bodies, and transformed into thought, which flits about, so to speak, becoming more and more brilliant, but at the same time more and more confused. Then the outer world disappears, and there remains only an inner world, sometimes full of tumult and delirium, and producing feverish excitement, or, as is more frequently the case, calm and quiet, and full of delightful repose. This intoxication is purely psychical, and far superior to the intoxication produced by alcohol or hasheesh, for, though hasheesh gives one a few hours of insanity, opium gives sleep, and with this boon there is nothing that can compare. One must have suffered from insomnia in order to appreciate the value of opium. It brings sleep, and it banishes pain.

It is one of the most powerful agents we possess for modifying the sensibility, but whether it does this by acting upon the sensor nerves or on the brain we know not with certainty. Even where it does not procure sleep, it has the singular power of calming the excitability of the nerves, and of subduing that morbid state of the sensibility called by physicians hyperæsthesia. It has been observed that when it reduces hyperæsthesia it does not cause sleep, all its force seemingly being spent in combating pain. In cases of stubborn neuralgia opium appeases suffering, and a larger dose is required to produce sleep. But is it not enough that it allays the irritability of a diseased nerve? Some persons cannot live without opium, and they swallow enormous quantities of it without perceptible effect. Herein opium differs widely from alcohol. Alcohol is cumulative in its effects, and the more one is addicted to its use, the more easily is he intoxicated by it. One does not become habituated to alcohol intoxication, but with opium the case is different; one may become so accustomed to it as to be able to drink daily a litre of laudanum, twenty drops of which would be a strong enough medicinal dose for a non-habituated person.

In China there is the same popular demand for opium that exists in Europe for alcohol and tobacco. The use of opium does not date very far back, and it is probably the only innovation that China has adopted from the West. The importation of opium from India into China amounted in 1798 to 300 tons, in 1863 to 3,000 tons, in 1866 to 3,903, and since then the increase has been still more rapid.

Opium is chewed, or smoked in a pipe, the latter mode of using it being the more common. The bowl of a long-stemmed pipe is filled with the drug, and, as the opium swells and adheres to the pipe, a needle is in constant use to keep open an air-passage. As the drug burns with difficulty, the smoker must have a light ready at hand for use whenever his pipe goes out.

The number of opium-smokers is considerable, but the great majority of them use the drug only in moderation. The wealthiest mandarins, the most intelligent merchants, smoke opium, as do the humblest coolies. The use of opium is like the use of tobacco among ourselves; nor does it produce any greater mischief, at least among the well-to-do classes; but with the common people it is different. There are establishments specially devoted to opium—smoking-places where, for a trifling sum of money, one may gratify this appetite. Rarely does a smoker leave before he is fully under the influence of the drug, just as the drunkard does not quit the gin-shop until he is fuddled. So used, opium is certainly a dangerous poison, and, according to the testimony of all travelers, the wretches who daily commit such excesses speedily fall to a fearful state of degradation, both moral and physical. Pale, wan, gaunt, shambling along with difficulty, they must have recourse to artificial stimulation in order to regain a part of their wasted energy. Still the injurious effects of opium have in all probability been very much exaggerated: the number of deaths caused by the abuse of the drug is not very great; and many of those who smoke it, even in considerable quantity, retain unimpaired their mental faculties. True, the digestive functions rarely escape impairment. Dyspepsia and general emaciation are the result of this sad habit; but, however that may be, China is not yet by any means on the brink of ruin, and, if she is in a state of decadence, the blame does not attach to opium.

Opium has its antidote: just as we can produce sleep, so too can we produce sleeplessness, by the employment of a mind-poison whose effects are diametrically opposite to those of the other. The antidote of opium is coffee. One hundred years ago coffee was almost unknown, but now there is hardly another beverage that is so widely distributed.

Everyone has it in his power to judge of the effects of coffee. For some persons it is a stimulus necessary for the performance of intellectual work. In others it produces a painful state of insomnia: taken even in weak doses it causes restlessness and anxiety, a sort of feverish activity altogether different from the indolent activity of opium. Under the action of opium the will seems to be lulled to sleep and the imagination runs riot. But under the influence of coffee the imagination is hardly stimulated at all, while there does appear to be excitation of the will. Did I not fear being suspected of having a theory to defend, I should say that the faculties of will and consciousness seem to be superexcited: there is, as it were, a constant strain on attention and memory, whereas in the case of alcohol, hasheesh, and opium, there is a relaxing of attention. Hence coffee produces a true intoxication that fatigues one far more than does the somnolent intoxication of opium, but it leads to the same result. In striving to do too much, the mind does less: under stimulation the will is impaired; and the perfect equilibrium of the mental faculties is disturbed as well by excess as by defect of will.

Coffee is said to produce cerebral anæmia, while opium and alcohol cause congestion; but this theory still needs confirmation. Nevertheless, the part played by coffee in general nutrition is very well understood. It retards organic combustion, and hence it is an *aliment d'epargne*—a food-stuff that effects a saving of other food-stuffs. In the normal state there is always going on within our tissues a multitude of chemical actions, the final result of which is heat-production and liberation of carbonic acid. This carbonic acid passes into the venous blood, and the venous blood, on reaching the lungs, parts with its carbonic acid. Thus the quantity of the carbonic acid is, to some extent, the expression of the nutritive activity. Now, on taking coffee, though no greater quantity of oxygen be inhaled, and without increasing the ration of food, the quantity of the carbonic acid is reduced, and yet the amount of force is not lessened. As illustrating this doctrine, it is usual to cite a fact observed among Belgian miners, who can perform a considerable amount of work almost without food, their strength being maintained solely by the absorption of a large quantity of coffee. Hence coffee is a food-stuff which moderates nutrition by lessening the activity of the chemical transformations incessantly going on within the tissues.